AMBULATORY MONITORING OF BLOOD PRESSURE: A GENERAL PRACTITIONERS' GUIDE

Dr Paul L Padfield

CONSULTANT PHYSICIAN / READER IN MEDICINE
DEPARTMENT OF MEDICINE
WESTERN GENERAL HOSPITAL
EDINBURGH

Doral House • 2(b) Manor

A NOTE ABOUT THE AUTHOR

Paul Padfield is a consultant physician at the Western General Hospital and a part-time reader in medicine at the University of Edinburgh. Qualifying from the University of Wales in 1970, his postgraduate training was completed in Glasgow and Ann Arbor, Michigan. His specialist activity is in endocrinology, and an interest in hypertension grew out of studies into salt and water metabolism while at the Medical Research Council's Blood Pressure Unit in Glasgow. Most recently, his work has involved research into the use of home and ambulatory monitoring of blood pressure, and he sits on the British Hypertension Society's working party on blood pressure measurement. He is author of many papers in the wide field of hypertension research, and has been active in Scotland in the production and audit of local guidelines for the management of hypertension.

ISBN

1 873839 06 5

Further copies of *Ambulatory monitoring of blood pressure: a GPs' guide* may be obtained from the Publisher, price £14.95 (ex. VAT). This publication reflects the view and experience of the author, and not necessarily those of the Publisher.

FOREWORD

Any new procedure or device which produces more efficient clinical management and patient benefits must surely be welcomed. If that procedure or device also provides us with cost benefits in these times of financial accountability, then it must be doubly welcomed.

Such a device is the 24-hour ambulatory blood pressure monitor. Its value is in the process of diagnosing new, suspected hypertension as well as in the follow-up of established hypertensive patients to assess whether or not treatment is beneficial. Classic methods of diagnosing hypertension are well known but, unfortunately, can be seriously flawed. This can result in erroneous diagnosis of raised blood pressure for a variety of reasons, one of the most important being 'white coat hypertension'. Such a diagnosis is not good for the patient, as he/she will be prescribed unnecessary drug therapy; neither is it good for the prescriber, for whom it will represent an unnecessary addition to an already over-burdened drug budget.

To obtain an accurate diagnosis of hypertension has its own obvious cost benefits. To assess further those patients who are maintained on antihypertensive therapy, and reappraise their status in relation to drug therapy and the avoidance of end-organ damage, is also an important part of efficiency in clinical care.

The advent of 24-hour ambulatory monitoring has helped clinicians worldwide to avoid the pitfalls of inaccurate diagnoses of hypertension, and a commitment to needless drug therapy for life. As its use spreads throughout all areas of both primary and secondary care, it will reduce the number of people put on unnecessary treatment, effecting a significant saving in the drugs bill.

For all of us in medical practice, whether or not we are fundholders, this workbook offers a way forward in the management of hypertension which allows for more efficient practice. I have no hesitation in recommending this book as an essential read to all in clinical care who need to manage hypertension and its sequelae.

Signed

D M . Tod.

David Tod
President, National Association
of Fundholding Practices

CONTENTS

GLOSSARY

AAMI	Association for the Advancement of Medical Instrumentation
ABPM	Ambulatory Blood Pressure Monitoring
ACE inhibitor	Angiotensin Converting Enzyme inhibitor
BP	Blood Pressure
DBP	Diastolic Blood Pressure
ECG	ElectroCardioGram
K-Sound	Korotkoff sound
LVH	Left Ventricular Hypertrophy
MRC	Medical Research Council
SBP	Systolic Blood Pressure
WHO	World Health Organisation

Chapter 1

MANAGEMENT OF HYPERTENSION

Hypertension, or raised blood pressure, is better regarded as a risk factor for cardiovascular disease than as an illness in its own right. This means that it falls into the same category as a raised plasma cholesterol, and, like this biochemical parameter, it usually produces no symptoms until a complication occurs. Therein lies the main dilemma for the doctor when faced with an individual with hypertension - treatment is designed to prevent ill health occurring, rather than to make the 'patient' feel better.

Managing hypertension, therefore, is a form of preventive medicine, and we need to be very clear that the risks of the condition are greater than those of treatment. All of this may be seem self-evident, but no form of intervention is without a potential for harm. Thus it behoves us, as clinicians, to be well aware of why we offer treatment to patients, and to be as precise as we can about the risks an individual may be subjected to over the next 10, 15 or even 20 years of his or her life.

Points to ponder

Reflecting on your previous clinical experience, how have you approached this dilemma?

In the field of cardiovascular medicine, doctors dealing with hypertension can reasonably afford to be confident. There are more randomised controlled trials demonstrating the efficacy, safety and long-term effects of drug treatment for hypertension than there are for most other disorders in medicine. In spite of the large body of evidence demonstrating that treating hypertension reduces cardiovascular events, however, we still have difficulty in deciding what to do with the patient who sits opposite us in our surgeries or clinics. The dilemma is not unique and will apply to any graded risk factor. An individual with a minor elevation of blood pressure will have a minor increase in risk, but a similar risk of any downside to treatment compared to the patient with, say, accelerated phase hypertension, who could be dead within six months without drug therapy.

When the Medical Research Council (MRC) published the results of its UK study of the treatment of mild hypertension in 1985[1], it provided convincing evidence that such treatment reduced the risk of stroke by approximately 40%. However, it demonstrated that to prevent one stroke, 850 people with mild hypertension (diastolic blood pressure 90-110 mmHg) would have to be treated for a year. The study showed no improvement in coronary artery disease event rates, and one wonders how many people of, say, 40 years of age, if offered such odds, would welcome life-long drug therapy, a 25-50% chance of needing two drugs to control hypertension and a 20% risk of noticeable side-effects?

Points to ponder

Consider your approach to putting an asymptomatic patient on a life-long therapy. How do you think you personally would cope if this happened to you?

The problem, of course, has been faced and the result is - 'guidelines'. It seems as if the past few years have seen the publication of an endless stream of advice on how to manage the patient with hypertension[2]. This would not be a problem if all advice were the same, but national and international bodies differ in the level of blood pressure above which treatment should be started, the importance of other risk factors in determining the treatment threshold, and the choice of drugs to use as first-line therapy.

The various guidelines all advise us to employ non-pharmacological means to lower blood pressure over a (variable) period of time, during which several measurements of blood pressure are made. The importance of this advice should not be underestimated. In the Australian National Blood Pressure study (published in 1980), almost half of the patients followed while on placebo therapy had a fall in blood pressure such that, after three years, they could no longer be said to have hypertension[3]. The situation was even more confusing in the above-mentioned MRC trial[1]. In this, 33-50% of patients on placebo were normotensive at their successive annual review measurements. However, these were not always the same people, so that a patient might have a diastolic blood pressure of 88 mmHg today, 98 mmHg next year and 86 mmHg the year after. As measurements in this study were much more carefully taken than they ever would be in 'the real world', it is plain to see how easy it would be to misclassify patients.

Perhaps we should look on a blood pressure measurement as having a sensitivity and specificity for predicting sustained hypertension. If, for example, we set a treatment cut-off point of 90 mmHg, we have a very sensitive test as virtually all patients with 'true hypertension' will be above this level; but it would be hopelessly non-specific as many, if not most, of the individuals at this level would then fall below the line on repeat measurement. The reverse would be true if we decided to treat at a diastolic blood pressure of 120 mmHg - the test would be virtually 100% specific, and thus we would hardly ever treat anyone inappropriately; the cost, however, would be a large proportion of people who could benefit from treatment being denied it (a low sensitivity).

The problem is thus a clear one, even if its solution may be difficult.

Doctors do not treat populations, they treat individuals, so what we need to devise is a strategy for targeting, as efficiently as we can, those patients who have most to gain from drug therapy while not treating those at a lesser risk. If treatment were always safe, we could adopt a more carefree, blunderbuss approach.

One of the messages to be taken from the various published guidelines is that the only solution to deciding who to treat, in the area of mild hypertension, is to amass a large number of measurements, over a period of time. It is, however, unclear whether one should use the average of all these measurements, the lowest value, or perhaps the value obtained at the end of a fixed period of monitoring, so it is difficult to see how the guidelines have helped us with this aspect of management.

Points to ponder

What guidelines do you adhere to? Have you an established practice policy? Do you think that your colleague in the next room adheres to the same management objectives that you do?

The fundamental principle in all this is the measurement of blood pressure itself. The standard mercury manometer, properly maintained, is potentially an accurate device. Those who use it are, however, prone to round off values to the nearest zero, to record either the muffling or the disappearance of sound as the diastolic blood pressure, and to vary the position of the patient on successive visits. It is not surprising then that the reproducibility of a clinic measurement of blood pressure is so poor, even before taking into account any true variability of the blood pressure itself.

Points to ponder

It has been recognised that precise blood pressure recording is dependent on efficient equipment. When did you last have your sphygmomanometer serviced and calibrated?

What if we had a device that could dispense with an observer, could measure blood pressure away from the potentially stressful environment of a doctor's surgery, could record multiple measurements of blood pressure, and was not subject to the same degree of variability as a clinic measurement. Assuming that such a device was 'user friendly', we would see it as a major advance; that is indeed what non-invasive ambulatory blood pressure monitoring is.

10

This workbook is designed to help the practising clinician to understand the limitations inherent in relying on standard measurement of blood pressure, while at the same time reminding him/her of the principles involved in identifying and targeting those at highest risk. Some aspects of risk stratification may be impracticable without the use of electronic blood pressure monitoring, while others are truly impossible without ambulatory devices. It would be disingenuous to suggest that any measurement of blood pressure will eliminate uncertainty in deciding what to do with patients on the borderline, but it will be suggested that the increased precision offered by non-invasive ambulatory blood pressure monitoring will better guide the clinician in the management of so-called benign essential hypertension.

Chapter 2

BLOOD PRESSURE MEASUREMENT AND DIAGNOSIS

DEFINITIONS

Blood pressure, like most biological variables, is uniformly distributed within a population such that there is no particular level of blood pressure (systolic or diastolic) that can be considered as a cut-off point separating normality from abnormality. The late Sir George Pickering spent most of his professional life defending this concept, and was fond of showing a series of blood pressure levels that at one time or other were considered to define hypertension. His comment was: *'They cannot all be right, and it is likely that they are all wrong'*. We do, however, need definitions so that we can learn to handle uncertainty (how can we manage hypertension if we cannot define it?), and thus there have come to exist some arbitrary cut-off points that are accepted by most authorities. The World Health Organisation (WHO) defines a normal blood pressure in subjects 18 years and above as a systolic of <130 and diastolic of <85 mmHg; high normal is 130-139 mmHg for systolic and 85-89 for diastolic. Hypertension is split into four stages:

- stage 1 (mild) - systolic 140-149, diastolic 90-99 mmHg;
- stage 2 (moderate) - 160-179/100-109 mmHg;
- stage 3 (severe) - 180-209/110-119 mmHg;
- stage 4 (very severe) - 210/120 mmHg or above.

A more pragmatic approach to defining hypertension would be to consider it to be that level of blood pressure above which intervention has been shown to improve outcome. As of 1994, this would mean 90 mmHg for diastolic and 160 mmHg for systolic, levels which take in a sizeable proportion of the population. It is important to remember that any level of blood pressure carries with it a risk that is greater than a slightly lower blood pressure.

Points to ponder

Take a moment to consider the ethnic and racial variation of raised blood pressure. What observations have you made?

In Western society, blood pressure increases with age, and this is particularly striking for the systolic blood pressure. We should not be lulled into thinking that this is a 'normal' phenomenon, however, as the absolute risk of a given blood pressure increases with age, so there is no argument for regarding hypertension as being less important in elderly people, or indeed for setting less rigid thresholds for intervention.

Given the problems of definition, it is perhaps not surprising that it is difficult to be precise about how common hypertension might be. Any answer would depend on the age of the population studied and the number of repeat measurements made, as well as the level of blood pressure taken to define abnormality. Nonetheless, it is likely that at least 10% of a middle-aged population will have sustained diastolic pressures above 90 mmHg. Above the age of 70 years, up to a quarter of the population might have a systolic pressure greater than 160 mmHg.

It is similarly difficult to decide to what level we should lower the pressure. Major benefits can be expected from any reduction in blood pressure, but most authorities set target blood pressures at which to aim. There would be no argument with a diastolic goal of 90 mmHg for all ages, and until recently a treatment goal of 140 mmHg for systolic pressure would have been accepted, even though there were no intervention trials to guide us. Now that specific intervention studies on systolic blood pressure have been completed (exclusively in the elderly) there are good data to support only a target of 160 mmHg. Following the argument that the lower the blood pressure the lower the risk of stroke, I would continue to argue for a goal of 140 mmHg, even in elderly patients, providing this can be achieved without undue side-effects.

VARIABILITY OF BLOOD PRESSURE

If we examine an intra-arterial record of blood pressure, it is clear that the levels vary continuously, minute by minute. Such a variation is superimposed on a major diurnal change, such that for some people the systolic pressure at night may be lower than the diastolic by day. Although there is still some argument as to whether this represents a true circadian rhythm, most would now accept that the differences can be best explained by a variable activity level. If an individual does not got to bed, then blood pressure does not fall; if he/she does go to bed, but does not sleep, then the day/night difference is less than when sleep occurs. The fall in blood pressure at night is of more than academic interest as those subjects with hypertension who do not show this may be at greater risk of the various forms of 'target organ damage' that appear to pre-date clinical events (one example is left ventricular hypertrophy). If this is to be an important aspect of blood pressure assessment for the future, then ambulatory monitoring will of course be essential.

The more commonly noted variation of blood pressure during the day has resulted in the term 'labile hypertension'. This term is seen as a barrier to decision-making only if the variability crosses the treatment threshold. A patient with a blood pressure of 160/100 mmHg on one day and 140/80 on another poses a more difficult management problem than the individual whose blood pressure moves from 160/100 to 180/120 mmHg, although both are equally labile. Multiple measurements will (if averaged) tend to smooth out these wide swings.

The most obvious form of labile hypertension has come to be known as 'white coat hypertension', and describes an individual whose blood pressure is elevated in the presence of a doctor or nurse, but normal in his/her own environment. Most individuals are subject to a white coat effect, but (as above) it only becomes a problem if the difference crosses our threshold for intervention.

Points to ponder

What measures could you take to avoid 'white coat hypertension'? In your opinion, could there be a difference between a doctor and a nurse in this effect?

Most blood pressures recorded as high initially will fall somewhat on repeated measurement. This in part reflects acclimatisation to the technique, but also a statistical phenomenon known as regression toward the mean (low blood pressures tend to rise on repeat). It should be manifestly clear, therefore, that a decision to embark on drug therapy ought to be based on a large number of readings rather than a few.

The advice of 'the guidelines' is based on studies such as those indicated in Chapter 1 of this workbook, which, by and large, indicate that the tendency for blood pressure levels to fall is complete (*for the group as a whole*) after four to six months. The risks of mild-to-moderate hypertension are not so dramatic for the individual, it is argued, that this period of time cannot be used to observe rather than to intervene.

The thrust of this argument is aimed at preventing inappropriate drug treatment for patients whose 'real' blood pressures are lower. But we should remember that we, as a profession, are not very good at ensuring that all who need treatment get it, and a potential pitfall of a long observation period is that some patients may be lost to follow-up. We do not know how common this might be in the UK, but in a recent French study some 10% of patients defaulted during a period when guidelines produced by the ISH/WHO were being followed[4]. It is likely that, without the resources of a controlled trial, the default rate might be greater still.

Points to ponder

Pause for a moment and think about the possible reasons for non-compliance with drug therapy and follow-up. By writing down your thoughts, you may be able to review your past and current practice.

Chapter 3

AMBULATORY BLOOD PRESSURE MONITORING

AMBULATORY MONITORS

At least a dozen devices are available for non-invasive ambulatory monitoring of blood pressure, and it is likely that many more will follow. All are expensive, but individual costs vary widely. Many, but not all, have been subjected to careful validation procedures; prospective users should therefore ensure that the equipment they intend to purchase has been properly validated, in accordance with the British Hypertension Society recommendations or the American guidelines issued by the Association for the Advancement of Medical Instrumentation(AAMI).

Points to ponder

Think about the outcome objectives that would be advantageous when considering investing in such a piece of equipment. Perhaps you could write these down and review your strategy.

OPERATION OF AMBULATORY MONITORS

All monitors consist of a central microprocessor, which can be preprogrammed to measure blood pressure at variable intervals throughout the period during which the monitor is worn (this can often be 24 hours). The monitor is connected to a cuff, which is inflated either by a small pump or a carbon dioxide cylinder. As with standard mercury manometers, the inflatable cuff comes in a variety of sizes to cover a range of upper-arm circumferences.

Most devices that employ an electric pump will require frequent battery changes, and not all of them accept rechargeable batteries. This can be an expensive running cost, as a set of four AA-type batteries may only be used reliably for two 24-hour periods with 30-minute inflations. Carbon dioxide cylinders have to be replaced at regular intervals, and should be supplied from the manufacturer as necessary.

For the measurement of blood pressure there are two techniques currently available.

Detection of Korotkoff sounds

Korotkoff sounds are detected by a microphone, which is either taped to the arm (with the cuff covering the microphone) or is integral to the cuff. For most users, this technology is quite familiar and easy to understand. However, devices incorporating the microphone within the cuff have inherent problems, particularly relating to movement, with the microphone moving away from the brachial artery during use. Moreover, a cuff with an integrated microphone is more difficult to clean, which can be an important drawback with continued use.

To improve accuracy, some monitors employ the technique of electrocardiogram (ECG) gating to ensure that the microphone genuinely detects a K-sound. An algorithm is devised such that only those sounds following the ECG complex by a predetermined interval will be recognised and recorded as K-sounds (Figure 1). Although there is some evidence to suggest that these devices may be more accurate (particularly where subject movement is concerned), positioning them on the patient can be time-consuming, they cannot be readily removed by the patient during use, and can give no readings if an ECG lead is loose. Modern devices will signal a fault if this happens, but a patient may be poorly prepared to cope with such circumstances.

We have seen at least one device that employs two microphones within the cuff. A K-sound is properly recognised if it passes from one microphone to the other. To allow better identification of K-sounds, some manufacturers have made major attempts to improve the software on these devices. The wave pattern of a K-sound is distinctive, but not necessarily unique to an individual. Increasing experience with this technology and further development of the software are likely to render the use of ECG gating unnecessary.

Oscillometry

Practitioners who have used small electronic devices for self-measurement of blood pressure will be familiar with this technology. The monitor detects the wave form in the artery. The first recognition of oscillometric waves determines systolic blood pressure, and maximum oscillations occur at mean arterial pressure. Devices by different manufacturers have unique algorithms to detect and record the diastolic blood pressure by calculation. However, manufacturers do not disclose how this calculation is derived, and this has been a source of irritation to some researchers. The monitors are extremely simple to apply as the positioning of the cuff is less critical than where a microphone is involved, and can even be applied over light clothing. Oscillometric devices are the most popular monitors throughout the world (Figure 2).

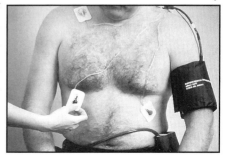

Data production

It should be noted that the monitors are better described as devices for multiple measurements of blood

Figure 1. A monitor measuring Korotkoff sounds and using ECG gating.

pressure in a normal environment, and are not truly ambulatory. Patients should always cease activity before blood pressure measurement, and most devices will give a warning sound which can be deactivated at night.

While it is not necessary for most practising clinicians to be familiar with what goes on inside the 'black box', it is important to know that all devices have built-in systems for discarding certain blood pressure readings. It is not always easy to identify the blood pressures

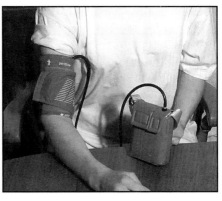

Figure 2. A oscillometric ambulatory monitoring device.

that the device will reject, but obvious errors, such as diastolic pressure exceeding the systolic or a zero for either reading, will be rejected. In assessing any blood pressure report, it is important to note how many readings are rejected, as a high rate of rejection (>10%) should cause some doubt as to the validity of the procedure.

Points to ponder

Before you read on, think about the frequency of measurements you might use with an ambulatory device and how long you might want a patient to wear it.

All monitors will allow the operator to pre-programme the interval of blood pressure recording. Moreover, patients can usually activate specific measurements at times of particular interest. There are no gold standards in determining the frequency of blood pressure measurement, but it is common to take measurements at half-hourly intervals. A recently published study which monitored more than 500 patients showed that the 'average' information obtained from 20-minute readings was the same as that for 10-minutes[5], and the choice of 30-minutes is a reasonable compromise for routine use. A large body of experience tells us that this practice is reasonably comfortable for patients, and does not in itself induce blood pressure elevation.

MONITORING PROCEDURES

It is common practice to apply the monitors for a full 24-hour period, thus obtaining approximately 48 recordings of blood pressure. When the machine is first applied, it is important to establish that a conventional measurement of blood pressure recorded simultaneously gives the same result as the electronic device. Most authorities would allow a difference of up to 5 mm for systolic and diastolic pressure at this time.

While the monitoring techniques are fairly easy to master, we should not underestimate the time it takes to learn to use ambulatory blood pressure devices correctly. There is also no doubt that the value of monitoring is enhanced by the input of a nurse or dedicated technician, in dealing with any problems that the patients might encounter in using the equipment.

When the device is returned by the patient, a report is generated. Reports from different devices vary slightly. There is usually a graphic demonstration of blood pressure throughout the period that the monitor is worn, together with a calculation of averages at preset time intervals. If the monitor is worn for 24 hours, there is usually an average blood pressure for that period, with separation of day and night times. One of the difficulties in interpreting 24-hour blood pressure data is the uncertainty over what should be regarded as 'day' and 'night'. Clearly, different information will be obtained if different time points are used, and it is therefore more consistent to record sleep and wake rather than any arbitrary clock time.

Another, as yet unresolved, dilemma relates to how one should handle the first few pressures recorded by the monitor while the patient is still with the nurse and in the hospital or surgery. As already discussed, this can be a time of particularly high pressure for some individuals. The more recordings made for comparison against a mercury sphygmomanometer for instance, the greater the effect on average blood pressure for that day. Potential solutions to this problem will be discussed later.

CLINICAL USAGE

Once the practitioner is confident that the monitor of choice will perform accurately, the next concern is knowing whether or not it will prove helpful in the management of patients and, if so, in which type of patient.

Points to ponder

Reflecting on the last few patients with hypertension that you have seen, when would you opt for 24-hour ambulatory monitoring and why?

It should be stressed that there have been no prospective studies of ambulatory monitoring of blood pressure used as the predictor of clinical outcome. There are, however, abundant data to indicate that target organ damage (heart, brain, retina, kidneys) can be better predicted by an ambulatory measure of blood pressure than any other measure taken in the clinical setting. Because of this, patients who are considered to be at small individual risk, particularly those with mild hypertension at the bottom end of the treatment range, are those whose management is likely to be influenced by their ambulatory pressures. Given that 70% of hypertensive individuals fall into the category of 'mild hypertension', such monitoring could present a considerable workload.

The British Hypertension Society has issued guidelines for a rather limited use of ambulatory monitors in clinical practice[6]. However, these guidelines suggest that the devices may be of help where 'white coat hypertension' is suspected. This phenomenon may affect at least 20% of patients with mild hypertension, and there is no way of predicting which individuals belong to this category without taking an actual measurement. In the US, recommendations for the use of ambulatory monitoring also include patients with apparently resistant hypertension, in whom there may be an element of the 'white coat' phenomenon.

Points to ponder

Could there be a variation in 'white coat hypertension', say, between regions in the UK, between countries or between different health-care delivery systems?

DATA ANALYSIS

Figure 3 outlines three typical traces, showing the type of information likely to be obtained from a 24-hour blood pressure profile. Clearly, any single reading within the 24-hour period may be unrepresentative of the whole. An average blood pressure over a specific length of time will smooth out what is essentially a discontinuous parameter. In general, therefore, individual spikes of blood pressure do not influence therapeutic decisions, and, as will be seen, it is the average over a given period that will determine what we do.

Points to ponder

Look at Figure 3 carefully, and examine what the three traces have in common and where they differ. What is your assessment of these three cases?

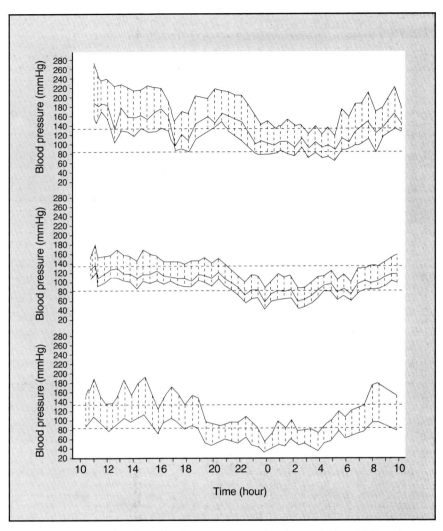

Figure 3. Three typical 24-hour blood pressure traces showing marked variability of pressure. Each trace demonstrates a major fall in blood pressure during the night with a rise on awakening the following morning. (Horizontal dotted lines represent the upper limit of normality for daytime systolic and diastolic blood pressure - 135/85 mmHg).

In the patient with 'white coat hypertension' (Figure 4), an average daytime pressure including the measurements made in the hospital/surgery may be artificially high, and it may be good practice to exclude such values from the calculation of the average. Some have advocated the application of monitors for 25 hours so as to allow the removal of the first hour and still have a '24-hour blood pressure'. While such an approach is almost certainly correct, it will involve more negotiations with manufacturers to alter their software if we are not to have to devise local systems for such corrections.

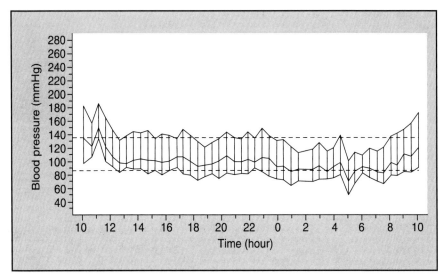

Figure 4. An example of 'white coat hypertension', where clinic blood pressures are high at the time the monitor is applied (left hand side of graph) and fall thereafter to near normal levels.

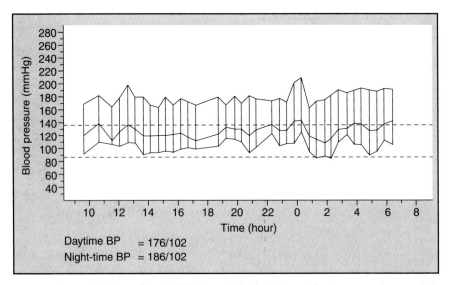

Figure 5. A so-called 'non-dipper'. This is an individual whose blood pressure does not fall during the night, and whose cardiovascular system is thus subjected to a more sustained blood pressure load.

The marked nocturnal fall in blood pressure seen in the three traces in Figure 3 has already been mentioned as being present in most individuals, whether hypertensive or normotensive. There is increasing information to suggest that patients whose blood pressure does not fall at night (Figure 5) may be at a greater risk of a wide range of target organ damage than those whose pressures do fall. This may well influence decision-making in an individual patient, for example if the average blood pressure during the day puts the individual on the borderline for drug treatment, a fall of less than 10% in blood pressure at night would be a factor to take into account in making therapeutic decisions.

If ambulatory pressure is measured in a large group of people and correlated against a clinic pressure, then it is possible to devise a formula for calculating the clinic pressure equivalent to a given ambulatory pressure. In a large study from Germany, this was calculated as a daytime ambulatory pressure of 135/85 mmHg being equivalent to a clinic reading of 140/90 mmHg[7]. In Edinburgh, taking a similar number of observations, we have shown that a clinic pressure of 140/90 mmHg is equivalent to a daytime ambulatory pressure of 136/86 mmHg (Figure 6).

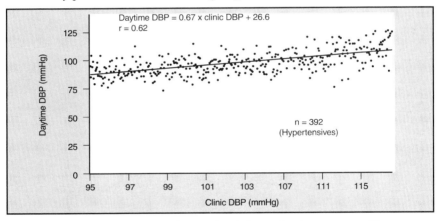

Figure 6. The relationship between clinic and ambulatory daytime pressure with a regression equation. It is possible to approximate one measurement knowing the other, but there remains a degree of scatter.

Points to ponder

During an average day (if such a thing exists), what variables may influence a person's blood pressure? How might these be taken into account?

Many authorities recommend the use of patient diaries to record activity, on the assumption that different levels of activity may influence blood pressure and thus alter the interpretation of results. It is certainly true that work blood pressures are higher than home blood pressures, but it is difficult to know how to take into account varying activity levels. To overcome this, many suggest that repeated measurements are taken in as similar fashion as possible, so that if monitoring is initially performed on a work day, it should be repeated under the same conditions. It is certainly the case that major discrepancies in activity will be highlighted by a diary, and should indicate caution in comparing successive monitorings. Perhaps one of the important uses of a diary is that it clearly shows when patients go to bed, so giving the best separation of day and night.

Points to ponder

So far, none of this has been very clinical. Take a moment or two to think about the patient using the ambulatory monitoring device. There are several day and night activities which could affect the readings or, indeed, affect the patient's comfort (and possibly compliance) at times. If you were that patient, how would you feel in that situation?

WHEN TO TREAT

For clinical purposes, what is required is a blood pressure figure that can be applied to determine whether drug therapy should or should not be employed. However, it is extremely unlikely that clinicians could ever afford to be dogmatic in this respect. Even in the more 'comfortable' area of clinic blood pressures, factors other than blood pressure have to be considered before drug therapy is decided upon.

Several population studies of ambulatory blood pressure are now available, which allow us to define 'normal' ranges. It is difficult, if not impossible, to apply such data to treatment thresholds, and we would often recommend drug therapy for patients whose blood pressure falls within the mathematically recognised definition of normality. It is probably safe to say that a daytime ambulatory blood pressure below 135/85 mmHg should be considered normal, whereas a blood pressure above 145/95 mmHg is high and should be treated. These figures apply to all age groups; there is no justification for applying different criteria in elderly patients. Within the grey zone, other risk factors will have to be taken into account in a management decision.

WHEN TO USE AMBULATORY MONITORING

Ambulatory monitoring offers two distinct advantages over any clinic measurement of blood pressure:

- Multiple measurements are obtained, smoothing out spontaneous variation, thus providing greater precision and reproducibility.
- Measurement of blood pressure away from an observer eliminates the 'white coat' effect. It may not be true to say that 'white coat hypertension' is entirely benign, but it is unequivocally less dangerous than sustained hypertension.

The council of perfection to my mind would indicate that all newly diagnosed hypertensive patients should have ambulatory monitoring performed. This is not yet practicable, although, as already indicated, patients with the mildest forms of hypertension, where most uncertainty exists, are those in whom the ambulatory monitor is likely to be most helpful. Table 1 indicates some of the situations which would have a broad measure of support for the use of these monitors.

Table 1. *Clinical situations where ambulatory blood pressure monitoring would be helpful*

- Patients with mild hypertension where a decision not to treat is being considered.
- Where a major difference exists between self-monitored blood pressure and clinic levels.
- Evaluation of resistant hypertension.
- Where the possibility of symptomatic hypotension arises.

Given the difficulties in identifying target blood pressures using ambulatory devices, it is more difficult to advocate their use for the long-term follow-up of patients with hypertension. If we believe, however, that an average daytime blood pressure of 140/90 mmHg is a more reliable measure than a similar clinic blood pressure, then this provides a reasonable target, with perhaps 135/85 for those with other cardiovascular risk factors.

DIFFICULTIES IN USAGE

We have monitored several thousand patients over the past seven or eight years, and there are very few in whom reliable recordings could not be obtained. There is good evidence that the repeated inflation of the cuff does not interfere greatly with the quality of sleep for most people and, even when it does, it has little effect on blood pressure. There is, however, a tiny percentage of patients who cannot tolerate the device. This cannot be predicted, so there are no patients who could not be offered the monitoring facility.

USE IN PRACTICE

One of the ongoing doubts in this area is whether such devices should still be reserved for the hospital centres or whether they should be used in general practice. We are still on a learning curve with the use of ambulatory blood pressure monitoring, and there are, as yet, too many unresolved issues to be able to recommend their unbridled use. At present, it seems most reasonable to argue that district hospitals should offer an ambulatory blood pressure monitoring facility to their local GPs in the same way that ECG services are available.

Chapter 4

MANAGING THE PATIENT

Ambulatory blood pressure monitoring should be part of a package of identifying the level of risk. We need to do all that is practicable in determining which patients require, or will benefit most from, antihypertensive drug treatment.

Points to ponder

Having arrived at this point in the workbook, has your opinion about the usefulness of ambulatory monitoring as an investigative tool changed in any way? If you have any doubts, why not list the advantages and disadvantages as you see them.

FURTHER INVESTIGATION

In the community, secondary hypertension is rare, and only those individuals with particular clues should be investigated with more than routine blood tests and urinalysis. There has been a suggestion, however,

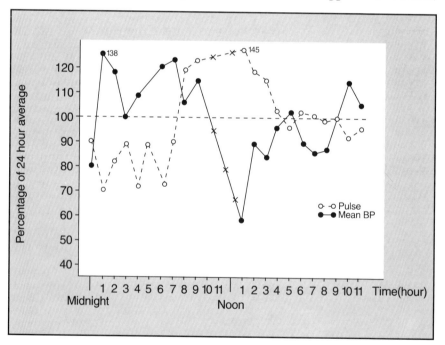

Figure 7. A patient with a phaeochromocytoma showing enormous swings in blood pressure, including a significant fall in blood pressure when the patient got out of bed during the night.

32

that ambulatory blood pressure monitoring may be helpful in identifying such patients. The individual with a phaeochromocytoma will characteristically exhibit wide swings in blood pressure, often with hypotensive episodes (Figure 7), and such a pattern is a justifiable reason for requesting measurement of urinary catecholamines or their metabolites.

Patients with other forms of secondary hypertension (particularly renal) are more likely to show a reduction in the normal nocturnal fall in blood pressure than are those patients with primary essential hypertension. Thus, it has been suggested that these patients should be targeted for further investigation. This is unrealistic; given that 15-20% of patients with essential hypertension may be termed 'non-dippers', even if all secondary hypertensive patients fell into the same category, a non-dipper would still be four times more likely to have essential hypertension (assuming a prevalence of secondary hypertension of 5%).

Points to ponder

What do you think are the other investigations that should be performed?

A dipstick urinalysis, plasma urea and electrolytes, cholesterol, and an ECG should be carried out. A chest X-ray is unhelpful in detecting left ventricular hypertrophy (LVH), and should not be requested routinely. An ECG can show specific changes of LVH, but it is very insensitive.

An echocardiogram is much more sensitive and can detect LVH in as many as 15% of patients with 'mild' hypertension. Such people are more likely to have an elevated ambulatory blood pressure, so there is no great likelihood of missing this important group of patients, who are at high risk, assuming a daytime blood pressure of less than 135/85 mmHg. It may however be important to consider an assessment of left ventricular mass in those whose ambulatory blood pressure is near 140/90 mmHg, as this is precisely the area where decision-making is most difficult. A normal left ventricular mass index in such a case would be reassuring, while an abnormal result (greater than $134g/m^2$ for men, $110g/m^2$ for women) would suggest the need for drug therapy.

If an echocardiogram were as simple to obtain and interpret as an ECG, we would perform this on all hypertensive patients. There are some who advocate that this should be done anyway as evidence of LVH on an echocardiogram would indicate the need for a more aggressive approach to the treatment of the raised blood pressure. This approach has enormous resource implications, but may develop. At the moment, we would only resort to an echocardiogram if faced with a patient whose clinic blood pressures dictate that he/she should be treated, but whose ambulatory pressures are normal or at least at a level that would not usually result in the introduction of drug treatment. Such an approach to the use of echocardiography may be more cost effective than its more widespread use.

It is traditional to measure plasma lipids in hypertensive patients as they are a 'high-risk' group. There does, however, remain some debate as to how much one should use an elevated plasma cholesterol as a factor in deciding whether to embark on antihypertensive therapy. An elevated plasma cholesterol is not a strong predictor for stroke, but it is for coronary heart disease. Unfortunately, the evidence that treatment of blood pressure reduces coronary heart disease events is not good, except for older patients, and thus it may not be correct to treat blood pressure more aggressively if cholesterol is high. This is a highly controversial area.

INITIATING DRUG THERAPY

The risks of symptomatic hypotension on first introducing a drug is small, and it is not justifiable to use ambulatory monitoring to check this. Some elderly patients have postural hypotension as well as supine hypertension, and it could well be helpful to look for adverse blood pressure effects early on in such people. Ambulatory monitoring would then be desirable.

FOLLOW-UP REQUIREMENTS

Twenty-four-hour control of blood pressure is taken to be a desirable goal of treatment.

Points to ponder

In your opinion, is this a reasonable intent?

It has already been indicated that 24-hour blood pressure is a better predictor of target organ damage and this presumably reflects the 'blood pressure load' on the system. Some researchers have used this concept to show that if blood pressure exceeds a given level for large proportions of the time, LVH is more likely to be present; that is, there is a high blood pressure load and more target organ damage. Such an observation is perhaps self-evident, as 24-hour blood pressure is in itself a better predictor of target organ damage. This does, however, allow another quantitative measure to be used.

While there are no prospective studies available to us that look at clinical outcome, one retrospective analysis of ambulatory monitoring performed at diagnosis of hypertension indicated that, for a given clinic blood pressure, those patients with a higher ambulatory blood pressure were more likely to suffer a cardiovascular event over a 10-year period. This study used only daytime pressures, as the monitors were not automatic. However, a persistently high blood pressure during sleep is also associated with a greater target organ damage, so 24-hour control is an important aim of antihypertensive therapy.

We need to be clear what we mean by this term, however, as it does not simply apply to the blood pressure measured just before the next dose of drug is taken. The value of ambulatory blood pressure monitoring lies in the reproducibility of an average produced from multiple measurements - there is less confidence in comparing two isolated

Points to ponder

Think about the characteristics of the antihypertensive agents that you have favoured in the control of blood pressure. Do you feel reassured that 24-hour control is achieved.

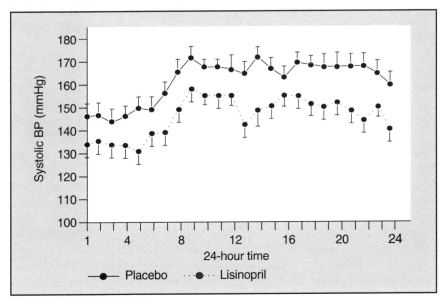

Figure 8. Effect on 24-hour blood pressure of a long-acting angiotensin-converting enzyme (ACE) inhibitor (lisinopril) given once-daily.

readings which could be done with a simple mercury manometer. Twenty-four-hour control, then, still refers to average blood pressure - the distinction is critically important.

It would be useful if we could vary therapeutic strategies to lower blood pressure preferentially at times when it is high (for example night-time in non-dippers), but little research has explored such an approach and most drugs, when given conventionally, will simply induce a parallel shift of the 24-hour profile (Figure 8).

It is, therefore, legitimate to monitor ambulatory blood pressure in patients on long-term drug therapy, and suggested goals have been indicated above.

Points to ponder

Because hypertension can be variable and may not, as previously thought, always be a life-long disorder, it may be pertinent at this time to review the guidelines in your clinical setting for the follow-up of such patients. The versatility of 24-hour ambulatory monitoring is clearly advantageous for the management of hypertension.

EXCESSIVE BLOOD PRESSURE REDUCTION

One possible use of ambulatory monitoring would be to ensure that blood pressure reduction is not too great. Again, a clinic blood pressure will only reflect one point in time and is unlikely to reflect the lowest blood pressure of the day (or night). There is a concern that excessive reduction of diastolic pressure might compromise coronary artery blood flow, particularly in those individuals with ischaemic heart disease or even LVH. It is also clear that some patients describe postural dizziness (particularly on waking), which might reflect excessive blood pressure reduction. The facility of blood pressure monitors to allow additional recordings when symptoms occur will enable the clinician to establish whether they relate to hypotension (Figure 9).

It must be said, however, that many older people have a surprisingly large fall in blood pressure at night (irrespective of drug therapy), and we must not necessarily assume that low nocturnal blood pressure is harmful (Figure 10). A degree of autonomic neuropathy is common in the elderly, and it may be difficult to deal with nocturnal hypertension without at the same time risking daytime or postural hypotension (Figure 9). Ambulatory monitoring of blood pressure makes such decisions easier.

Overall, the benefits of ambulatory blood pressure monitoring in the management of chronic hypertension are the same as those at diagnosis - it is more reproducible, and thus reliable, than a clinic blood pressure.

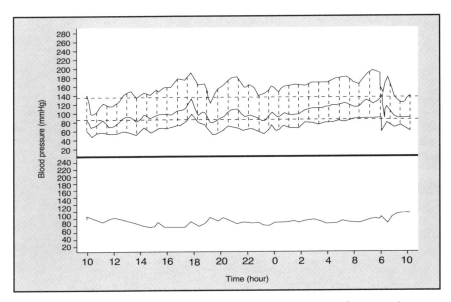

Figure 9. Twenty-four-hour ambulatory blood pressure in a patient with autonomic neuropathy, showing significant hypertension at night but low blood pressure causing hypotensive symptoms during the day.

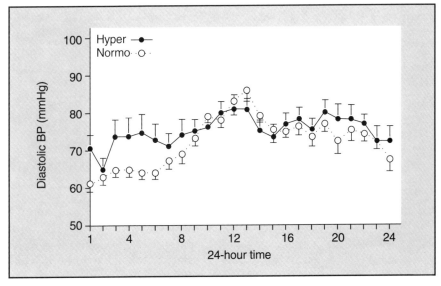

Figure 10. A comparison of 24-hour blood pressure in two groups of elderly patients, one receiving antihypertensive treatment, and the other not. Both groups had similar clinic blood pressures, and it can be seen that the tendency for blood pressure to fall during the night is, if anything, greater in those patients not receiving antihypertensive therapy.

NON-DRUG MANAGEMENT

This has been touched upon already, and nobody doubts that reductions in calorie, alcohol and sodium intake should form part of all antihypertensive strategies. Many patients with the mildest form of blood pressure elevations can be managed without drug therapy, but it is not clear how well compliance can be maintained over many years. An annual monitoring of ambulatory pressure would be perfectly appropriate for such patients who, by the very nature of their blood pressure elevation, are at low individual risk (Figure 11).

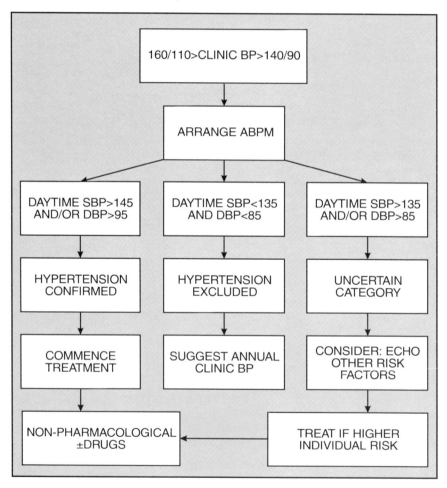

Figure 11. Flow diagram for the suggested use of ambulatory blood pressure monitoring in the assessment of patients with mild hypertension. In any patient, evidence of target organ damage would necessitate treatment.

REFERENCES

1. Medical Research Council Working Party. Trial of treatment of mild hypertension: principal results. *Br Med J* 1985; **291**: 97-104.
2. Swales JD. Guidelines on guidelines. *J Hypertens* 1993; **11**: 899-903.
3. Report by the Management Committee. The Australian Therapeutic Trial in mild hypertension. *Lancet* 1980; **i**: 1261-7.
4. Chatellier G, Battaglia C, Pagny JY, *et al*. Decision to treat mild hypertension after assessment by ambulatory monitoring and World Health Organisation recommendations. *Br Med J* 1992; **305**: 1062-6.
5. Palatini P, Mormino P, Canali C, *et al*. Factors affecting ambulatory blood pressure reproducibility. *Hypertension* 1994; **23**: 211-6.
6. Sever P, Beevers G, Bulpitt C, *et al*. Management guidelines in essential hypertension: report of the second working party of the British Hypertension Society. *Br Med J* 1993; **306**: 983-7.
7. Baumgart P, Walger P, Jurgens U, *et al*. Reference data for ambulatory blood pressure monitoring: what results are equivalent to the established limits of office blood pressure? *Klin Wochenschr* 1990: 723-7.

SUGGESTED READING

Appel LJ, Stason WB. Ambulatory blood pressure monitoring and blood pressure self measurement in the diagnosis and management of hypertension. *Annals Internal Med* 1993; **118**: 867-82.

Middeke M, Schrader J. Nocturnal blood pressure in normotensive subjects and those with white coat, primary, and secondary hypertension. *Br Med J* 1994; **308**: 630-2.

Palantini P, Mormino P, Canali C, Santonastaso M, De Venuto G, Zanata G, Pessina AC. Factors affecting ambulatory blood pressure reproducibility. *Hyperten* 1994; **23**: 211-6.

Pickering T. Third International Symposium on Ambulatory Blood Pressure Monitoring. *Amer J Hyperten* 1993; **6.**

Stewart MJ, Padfield PL. Blood pressure measurement: an epitaph for the mercury sphygmomanometer? *Clin Sci* 1992; **83**: 1-12.

Stewart MJ, Padfield PL. Measurement of blood pressure in the technological age. *Br Med Bull* 1994; **50**: 420-42.

PRACTICE POINTS

Cost-effectiveness

It is still commonplace for patients to be started on antihypertensive therapy after only two or three blood pressure recordings, and thus it remains likely that some patients may be treated unnecessarily with drugs. Evidence in support of this comes from withdrawal studies where up to a quarter of patients stopping antihypertensive drugs remain normotensive for at least a year - some of these patients probably never had sustained hypertension. While it is true that a rigorous adherence to guidelines (for the identification of patients with mild hypertension) will target the correct proportion of patients needing therapy, such an approach requires repeated visits for re-checking of blood pressure. This is costly for both doctor and patient, and some patients may be lost to follow-up. It has been calculated in the US that by eliminating 'white coat hypertension', a decision based on ambulatory monitoring will reduce the number of patients put onto life-long drug therapy, reduce surgery visits, and thus pay for itself in a very short time. Ambulatory monitoring identifies a similar proportion of patients for therapy as does a careful following of the ISH/WHO guidelines.

Patient education

The statistic that we need to treat 850 people with mild hypertension for one year to prevent one stroke[1] makes it difficult to recommend drug therapy for all of the asymptomatic people who are found to have a diastolic blood pressure above 90 mmHg. Most patients can easily grasp the concept of total blood pressure load or burden, and it may thus be easier to convince them of the need for treatment if they can be shown the graph of their own blood pressure over a day and night, in their own environment. The idea that the average blood pressure over time is a better predictor of risk is, in my experience, easily understood and is helpful in persuading patients of the need for drug therapy. It also teaches them (and us) to be wary of over-interpretation of single blood pressure readings.

Doctor education

All doctors using ambulatory blood pressure monitoring should wear the monitor for at least one 24-hour period. This allows them to speak with confidence when describing the technique to a patient. It is likely to be far more convincing for a patient if a doctor can indicate that he/she slept well while wearing the monitor.

The role of the nurse

The practice nurse should play a critical role in the initial assessment and follow-up of hypertensive (or possibly hypertensive) patients. Nurses induce a smaller 'white coat' effect, and generally take more time to explain things to patients. Patients may be more prepared to ask questions of a nurse than of a doctor; thus it is critical that practice nurses become educated in all facets of measurement and treatment of hypertension. The British Hypertension Society has a branch for nurses, and if a practice nurse is designated to devote a lot of time to this area, it would be prudent for him/her to join. The nurse will be conversant with the ambulatory monitoring and also with whatever self-monitoring the practice might use. It is my experience that the nurse will rapidly become much better acquainted with the techniques than many doctors.

PATIENT PROFILES

Patient 1

A 54-year-old man was persuaded by his wife to attend a well-man clinic where his blood pressure was recorded as 168/102 mmHg.

He had no other risk factors for cardiovascular disease, and did not admit to being anxious about his blood pressure.

An ECG and routine blood and urine tests were normal, and the practice nurse loaned him a small electronic sphygmomanometer for a week. During this time he measured his blood pressure about 12 times, but all readings were taken at home as he had been reluctant to take the machine to his work (he was employed as a solicitor's clerk). At home, his blood pressure varied from 122/76 to 158/96 with an average of 140/88 mmHg.

His doctor referred him to hospital for an ambulatory blood pressure recording. He tolerated the device and was surprised at how little it affected his work or sleep. The hospital reported that the average daytime blood pressure was 138/86 mmHg, falling to 126/78 at night.

The advice to the GP was to arrange for annual checks of blood pressure, but not to initiate drug therapy.

Comments

There is no doubt that this man is on the border-line of needing drug therapy, and an echocardiogram might be considered if a repeat ambulatory blood pressure a year later is any higher. Such patients are at low risk, but need continued follow-up.

Patient 2

A 62-year-old obese woman presented to her GP with a headache. The doctor noticed that there was no blood pressure recorded in her case notes, but the patient recalled that her blood pressure had been high during both of her pregnancies. Blood pressure was recorded at 178/108 mmHg and she appeared anxious.

She was referred to the practice nurse for repeat measurement of blood pressure, but defaulted after a further two visits where blood pressure had been 152/86 and 146/90 mmHg.

Two years later she fell, sustaining a left Colles' fracture, and was noted by the casualty officer to have a blood pressure of 200/110 mmHg.

The GP then referred the woman to a hypertension clinic with a specific request for ambulatory monitoring, as he thought she might have 'white coat' hypertension.

An ambulatory monitor was fitted, and the blood pressure at the time of fitting was 168/108 mmHg and 176/106 on repeat. It fell thereafter, but her average daytime pressure was 146/94 with a night-time pressure of 128/86 mmHg.

She was told that she was unequivocally hypertensive and advised to lose weight. She was unsuccessful over two months and bendrofluazide 2.5 mg was started.

Comments

This patient has a pronounced 'white coat' effect, but still has hypertension. Calorie restriction should lower blood pressure, but as is often the case the patient could not manage this. Long-term follow-up may be difficult without the use of ambulatory monitoring.

Patient 3

A 56-year-old man had been attending his GP for five years for treatment of his blood pressure. He had been tried on several different drugs and most had either proved ineffective or side-effects had been severe.

At the time of referral to the hospital he was taking amlodipine 10 mg, enalapril 20 mg and frusemide 40 mg, and his most recent blood pressure readings were 168/100 and 178/110 mmHg. He stated that he was 100% compliant as he took all three tablets at breakfast.

There were no other cardiovascular risk factors, and no evidence of target organ damage was noted on routine testing.

At the time the ambulatory monitoring was fitted in hospital, his blood pressure was 176/106 mmHg. For the rest of the day, his average pressure was 138/80 mmHg and at night 126/74.

An echocardiogram was arranged, and this showed no evidence of left ventricular hypertrophy.

Comments

This man has 'white coat' hypertension, and his apparent resistance to drugs represents the typical, non-habituating, pattern of this condition.

At this point in time, it is unclear how much drug therapy he needs and a careful back-titration with ambulatory monitoring would be reasonable.

He requires life-long follow-up.

Patient 4

A 48-year-old slim woman was prompted to attend her GP after experiencing attacks of excess perspiration for no good reason. She thought it was the menopause and wished to discuss hormone replacement therapy.

Her GP recorded her blood pressure at 218/122 mmHg with no clinical evidence of target organ damage. Urinalysis was negative, but an ECG recorded at that visit showed evidence of left ventricular hypertrophy. The GP had been loaned an ambulatory monitor by a pharmaceutical company, and he fitted the machine there and then asking the patient to return the next day.

The blood pressure profile was striking in that there were enormous swings of blood pressure (see Figure 7), and the average during the day (186/110) was less then that at night (194/116). The GP surprised the local hospital by referring the patient with a diagnosis of phaeochromocytoma.

Comments

The 24-hour profile is typical of phaeochromocytoma. A loss of diurnal rhythm is seen more frequently in secondary forms of hypertension (mostly renal), but, unless the nocturnal blood pressure is actually higher than that during the day, essential hypertension is still more likely even in a 'non-dipper'. If a patient sleeps badly while wearing the monitor, this might be an explanation for a higher pressure during the night.

Patient 5

A 44-year-old male business executive was found at an insurance medical to have a blood pressure of 150/100 mmHg. He was an active man, played squash twice a week and led a 'stressful' professional life. His father (aged 74 years) had been on treatment for hypertension for 10 years. The patient had no complaints and felt well. He was reluctant to take drug therapy. His GP had advised non-pharmacological approaches with a reduction in sodium and alcohol intake. After six months his blood pressure was still high varying between 146/98 and 152/104 mmHg.

He was referred for ambulatory monitoring. There was little or no 'white coat' effect as his blood pressure at the time the monitor was put on was 156/106 mmHg, and his average daytime pressure was 148/100. After being shown the blood pressure trace he accepted the need for antihypertensive therapy and was started on atenolol 50 mg/day.

An echocardiogram showed no evidence of left ventricular hypertrophy, and he was not advised to stop playing squash.

Comments

This is quite a common problem. His elevated ambulatory pressure dictates the need for medical therapy. Stories of sudden death while playing squash make one concerned about such strenuous activity, but the lack of left ventricular hypertrophy is reassuring.

Patient 6

A 48-year-old female school teacher, who found her work particularly stressful, attended her GP as she was not sleeping well. She had no risk factors for cardiovascular disease, but her blood pressure was 158/104 mmHg and tended to be high on repeated measurement. She was given an electronic self-monitoring device which she took to school. She noticed that her blood pressure was often high while at school, but usually less than 140/90 mmHg at home or at weekends.

She was referred to the hypertension clinic, and wore an ambulatory monitor on two occasions - midweek and on a Sunday.

Her pressures revealed that during the week her daytime pressure was 148/95 mmHg falling to 138/80 at night. On the Sunday, her daytime pressure was normal at 134/85 mmHg falling to 128/80 at night.

An echocardiogram showed no evidence of left ventricular hypertrophy, and she was given no antihypertensive treatment. She was referred to a psychologist for relaxation therapy.

Comments

This illustrates one of the difficulties of ambulatory monitoring - we have more information than we know what to do with. Her blood pressure is high enough to warrant treatment when she is at work, but not when she is away from school. Her clinic blood pressure would dictate drug therapy, but the approach of trying to deal with her stressful life without drugs is important. A clinic blood pressure would not give us enough information in this particular patient.

Patient 7

A 76-year-old man had been followed by his GP for several years with systolic hypertension. The GP had numerous readings in the region of 180/80 mmHg.

The patient was well, was on no regular medication and appeared to have no other cardiovascular risk factors. As a result of attending a local meeting on hypertension in the elderly, the GP thought that the patient required drug therapy, so she referred him to the hypertension clinic for further assessment.

The hospital recorded similar levels of blood pressure and arranged an ambulatory monitor. The daytime average was 138/76 mmHg, with a night-time pressure of 136/73. An ECG and subsequent echocardiogram revealed no evidence of left ventricular hypertrophy. A recommendation to start bendrofluazide 2.5 mg was made.

Comments

This is the most difficult aspect of decision-making with ambulatory monitoring of blood pressure - the patient who has a major discrepancy between the clinic and ambulatory readings. There is some suggestion in the literature that 'white coat hypertension' is more common among patients with isolated systolic hypertension, but which blood pressure represents the true state of affairs? The trial data dictate that the patient requires drug therapy, and the physician responsible was not happy to ignore the sustained clinic hypertension, in spite of the lack of target organ damage.

It is difficult to be dogmatic in such a situation, and clearly the decision to stay with trial data is hard to fault. We have elected not to treat several younger patients in a similar situation with both systolic and diastolic hypertension, and I know that this is the case with many colleagues throughout the world. If one elects not to treat an unequivocally raised clinic level on the basis on a normal ambulatory pressure then clearly follow-up is important.

Patient 8

A 30-year-old woman was referred by her GP after requesting an oral contraceptive agent. Her blood pressure on two occasions was 152/94 and 164/92 mmHg. There was nothing else discovered on history or examination, and the routine investigation results were normal.

She reluctantly agreed to wear an ambulatory monitor, and was seen again at the clinic the following week. At the time the monitor was fitted her blood pressure was 158/98 mmHg, and at the second visit it was 146/94. She complained about the monitor, saying it was painful and kept her awake at night. There were many gaps in her 24-hour record, although the average of those values obtained was 152/88 mmHg.

She refused to repeat the measurement and defaulted from the hospital clinic. The GP has since started her on a calcium antagonist as her blood pressure remained elevated.

Comments

In my experience, less than 1% of patients find the monitor intolerable and less than 5% complain of problems at night. Most patients are aware of some inflations during the night, but there is good evidence that for most this does not interfere with the recording obtained. It was suspected that this particular patient may have removed the monitor at various times and any reading which has more than 10% of readings not made must be suspect.

Patient 9

A young man aged 35 years attended an insurance medical. His blood pressure was recorded at 164/98 mmHg, but he had no other risk factors for cardiovascular disease. His blood pressure was measured again after five to 10 minutes of rest and again it was high at 158/96.

His GP recorded similar readings at the surgery, but a daytime ambulatory monitored blood pressure was significantly lower at 134/80 mmHg. At the time the monitor was fitted, his reading was 162/90 - a marked 'white coat' effect.

On the strength of the ambulatory monitoring readings, the insurance company did not load his policy and he obtained life cover.

Comments

Life insurance companies are able to calculate the risk of premature death with a good deal of precision, and it was noteworthy that we were able to persuade them of the validity of a normal blood pressure via ambulatory monitoring by quoting data on surrogate markers of morbidity and mortality.

I am not sure that all companies would respond in the same way, however; in another recent case ambulatory monitoring was not accepted!

Patient 10

A 19-year-old medical student found that her blood pressure was 148/92 mmHg during a physiology practical. She knew that both her parents had hypertension, so she went along to her family doctor who recorded readings of 148/90, 144/94, 146/92 and 140/94 over a four-week period.

The GP had been loaned a 24-hour monitor and the student wore this, recording a daytime average of 136/88 mmHg with 122/80 at night. The GP telephoned the hospital for advice.

After discussion, the advice given was for the student to reduce her sodium intake and to continue regular exercise. Her GP would follow her blood pressure but would not introduce drug therapy.

Comments

There seems little doubt that this woman is hypertensive, and apart from supporting the clinic diagnosis, ambulatory monitoring has not added much. The argument that we do not know at what level of ambulatory blood pressure we should introduce drug therapy applies equally well to clinic blood pressure at this age. Although there are some normative data for ambulatory blood pressure in young people, it is even more difficult to know at what level drug therapy should be instituted.

The life-time risk for this young woman may be significant, but her individual risk over the next few years is small, and an expectant approach is justified.

INDEX